Dedication

I dedicate this to the many women whose lives were cut short by a cancer they have been dealt. I thought about naming a few but there are too many and someone would be left out. Some I have met in person, most have been through three ovarian cancer sites on the internet (only one today is still active and for that I am eternally grateful) Yet, I can't separate these lives from those who are still fighting the fight. The guidance I received and the friendships created are more intense because of the journey we share. You are all at the forefront of my mind. This story belongs to you all.

I dedicate this also to family, friends and colleagues. You are there for me in too many ways to count. You are my rock and time with you remains my goal.

And to the medical teams: the doctors, the nurses, the lab techs, the pharmacists, the receptionists, the assistants and every person who impacts the ride, I couldn't make the trip without you.

To save one life is to save the world and I hope somehow my journey will have the ability to help someone at some time and some place.

D1522371

Prologue

I am part of the class of 2007. That means I am approaching ten years.

I've learned so much along the way and have had so many people tell me I should write it down. I have always hated writing and felt I am not very good at it.   Things changed when I wrote part of a weekly column called "Friday's Corner". This column was written by a member known as 'rabbitgirl' on the *Team Inspire* site. Her writings each week were informative, technical, emotional and sometimes just plain funny. After she passed away we were all saddened immensely, but decided to continue the column in her memory We each signed up for a different week. I learned something when I sat down to write my column. The words just flowed. The feedback made me realize I had a lot of important information to pass on.

So, it may not be all or part of a column or it may be a self-made storybook of a journey. I hope to convey what I learned and how that information can help others, and not just those with ovarian cancer. I believe much of this information can be translated to a multitude of cancers.

Just some basic information that I think you should know about me which probably won't come up early on in the journey but might be helpful in following. I am 62 years young and am married to a wonderful man for just over ten years. Between us we have six children (and four amazing daughters-in-law and a son in law) And the best of the best.... six granddaughters, four of whom have been born since diagnosis.

I have an amazing full time job as the executive director of a women's nonprofit with phenomenal volunteers, staff and colleagues. All could not be more supportive as I go through many different trials and treatments. I have worked straight through this process.

And medically, which we know is crucial, I have a team of doctors, nurses, general staff and lab techs stretching from my main hospital RWJBarnabas in Livingston New Jersey, to Dana Farber in Boston, U Penn in Philadelphia, NYU and Sloan Kettering in New York. Living in the northeast provides excellent opportunities.

And finally I have a lot of luck. Some people believe in faith during the process, for me I just simply consider myself lucky.

I plan on living with cancer a lot longer and with the information and support I have, I hope to continue to own it.

I did not write this to be a memoir of my experience. Over time people knew how much I had learned and suggested I write it down   When I read it back it sometimes seems a little too much like just my story. I don't know how to do it differently. I truly have one goal; that one thought, that one section or one piece will help someone else get through a day just a little bit easier.

In the beginning

Some things seem so clear even though they happened almost ten years ago. Life was good. My daughter was a senior in high school, her field hockey team had just won the state championship (again). She was headed to an amazing college with a field hockey scholarship. My two oldest had graduated from college, one working and one at grad school. And my third was still in college. I was married to a wonderful man and we were approaching our first anniversary. (Most people I know say that for me third time was the charm).

We had a busy time around Thanksgiving and were heading to California for a field hockey tournament. I was sick as a dog. When we got to the hotel with two of my kids I said I needed to go to the emergency room. In short order I was diagnosed with a urinary tract infection and given antibiotics. I did make it to every game (always have to set priorities) but didn't eat much and didn't feel better. By the time we got home I was feeling a little better, but not perfect. Then I got a cold and ran out of the antibiotics. So, I made an appointment to see a new internist. He gave me a new antibiotic prescription and suggested I make an appointment with my gastro doctor based on my history of colitis. Right before I left his office he mentioned maybe I should plan on a CT scan as well.

I made one appointment with the gastro doctor and another one for the scan. My gastro doctor, wanted to see what the scan showed. So on a Thursday morning I went for the scan. I asked when I should get the results (always ask) and he said with the weekend coming probably Monday or Tuesday. Not happy, but understandable. Patience is not my forte.

Went home, had lunch. Less than two hours after the scan I got a call from the doctor's office. There is a mass on the ovary and I should make an appointment with my gynecologist. It was starting to snow when I called their office. They said my doctor was done with appointments for the day and someone would call me after they received the fax.

My husband and I had a quick discussion. His wife had passed away from breast cancer three years earlier and this was no joke. Since my internist's office is across the street from my gynecologist's we got into the car and went and picked up the report. Hell yes, this was going to be in our control, not a wait and see game.

Went across the street and demanded to see a doctor with fax in hand. Turns out my doctor was still in the office. Lesson #2 ask directly when you call an office not just for an appointment, but to talk to your doctor when it is important. (By the way actually, lesson #1 was not waiting for any damn fax machine to run my life). So the doctor did an exam and felt something. He did a ca125 blood test right in his office and then called to make me an appointment for a vaginal ultrasound. Yea for all the snow coming down. Lots of cancellations. Got my gallon of water to drink and went to the office. Lab techs really don't give you many hints even though I tried. Friday morning came and I called my gynecologist. Oh yes, a few times…. He said results were not in yet but he would call as soon as he had them. At 1pm I got the call. First thing he says is that he already made me an appointment with a gynecological oncologist for Tuesday. Already that didn't sound good. Ironically he didn't give me ca125 results, and I didn't ask. That would never happen again. So now we had a whole weekend plus a day to wait. Ugh. He also told me to be careful what we read on the internet. Good suggestion.

Then I wondered, why did I have to wait for Tuesday. I wanted a Monday appointment. Even though he had more clout than me, I decided to call the office. Well I actually had the earliest appointment since the doctor was in surgery on Fridays and Mondays. So Tuesday it was.

We did spend the weekend doing some research, mainly about the doctor. We loved his credentials. Also did some research about ovarian cancer. Got a sense of ca125 numbers and the staging aspects. Tried to stay away from the grim stuff. Not my nature.

Tuesday came and we loved the doctor. He explained about ca125s and false negatives. The highest false negative he had seen was 700. Reality here, mine was 1400. We needed to do surgery and see what there was to see. Lucky me! He had an opening in three days on

December 21st, holiday weekend. Otherwise we would have to wait till after New Year's. Hell, no!

So, surgery goes pretty much as expected. I am an optimist, but also a realist. Thinking 1400 was too high for nothing I had a sense it was really going to be about staging. When I woke up I got the news with my husband. They removed my ovaries, other paraphernalia and also tumors in abdomen and pelvis. Probably stage 3 but would have to wait. He said he got 80% out. I think that was when I freaked a little. Why not 100%? He explained that in his experience rather than be more invasive and do substantive damage, he got what was easily removable. Then we would do three treatments of frontline chemo, then a second surgery when much of it might be gone and then three more treatments. Ok then. Just to jump ahead here, before the second surgery my ca125 was down to 35 and after the surgery he said that about 18% of the 20% was gone due to chemo. Good plan then. Loving my surgeon.

Back to diagnosis weekend. On Saturday the covering oncologist comes in. Not someone my husband already knew, but after all it was Christmas weekend and he was the Jewish doctor on staff. I was pretty good with that, being Silverman myself. He spent about two hours with us and we made a decision based upon the surgery. Since the surgery wasn't too invasive I would start chemo on December 31st. One week away. Let's do it. We also had a two-hour appointment in his office. I learned that he is very good at drawing. He drew what he was talking about so we could picture. He also drew the differences between how breast cancer works as opposed to ovarian. That was important because of my husband's experience. Since my husband was familiar with other doctors at the hospital I asked him what he thought. Turns out we were both sold on Dr. G. And so the journey began ....

One note on what not to do after abdominal surgery. Do not play bingo at the hospital with your four kids when the men running it on the TV were a little funny… ok alot funny. My kids had me hysterical laughing. And laughing really hurts after abdominal surgery.

Family History: Past, present and future

During the week I was home before chemo I thought about lots of questions. My mom and I discussed the fact that my father had six sisters, three who died in their 60s. We knew there was some cancer but no one talked about the "C" word in those days. So, we called some of my cousins. Not a real surprise here. One aunt died from heart disease, one had ovarian cancer and one had ovarian and breast cancer. Kind of left me feeling pretty sure I had the BRCA gene. If I had only known this in advance I might have saved myself this diagnosis and cancer. My gynecologist had already spoken to me to ask about any history. I decided then that I needed to be tested but testing would have to wait until after I finished treatment. One thing at a time. Nothing was going to change my current status.

I finished frontline treatment in July and the following week went to the geneticist. The process took longer than I would have liked. It was frustrating. I knew what the results were going to be but they wouldn't even do the test until I did paperwork and survey. Finally, at the second or third appointment they did the blood work. Again, I was told it would take two to three weeks. Ugh, I hate waiting. After two weeks I remember calling her to check in. I was at the beach.

She said that she just got the results but I had to make an appointment and there was no availability for two more weeks. Notice a theme here: Not happening!! I asked her to please give me the results over the phone. The survey had shown I had a 99% risk of being BRCA positive. She said she has never done that before. Her policy is that she gives all results in person. I explained this was a good first time. After all, I just finished six months of chemo. I have cancer, this is not preventative counseling. After a lot of prodding she finally said yes you are BRCA 1 positive. Again and we will discuss this later... be your own best advocate. I have the 187delg mutation. Ok then, no surprises but the next move was to find a breast surgeon. When faced with the stats – a 47% risk of ovarian cancer, which I have, and an 87% risk of breast cancer, I wanted them babies gone. One cancer is plenty for me. It was not a matter of what treatment to do, it was a question of the type of prophylactic mastectomy, the reconstruction and the doctor. Oh, and of course if that wasn't enough, you have to figure in insurance approvals. By the end of the weekend I was pretty clear which procedure and which doctors. For the Internet we must be eternally grateful. In the end I was able to meet with the doctors, get insurance approved, and make the decision to wait six months to allow my body to recover from the chemo. I also decided to increase my breast size just a bit. Why not? In terms of the procedure it was all done in one step. Removal and implants all in one day. Best decision for me.

"Force" is a tremendous resource for BRCA positive women or men. (Remember I got this from my father). It is an organization focused on BRCA. Use it or recommend it. And make sure at some point your children get tested.

I truly hadn't planned on my daughter getting tested at age 22 while still in college. Her decision to get tested was based on the fact that my daughter-in-law's sister at age 28 was diagnosed with breast cancer. Turned out she had the BRCA gene and a family history of ovarian cancer (I knew about the ovarian cancer from her father and had suggested testing). Again, I believe knowledge is a gift. She had her surgery and reconstruction. My daughter-in-law was negative but her other sister was also positive. She had the prophylactic surgery and reconstruction as well. This truly brought things home to my daughter. She decided at that point she wanted to know. When she was home in October that year, she got tested. Got results over Thanksgiving and then over Christmas break did her surgery. In the twenty-four hours after the results she evaluated the different procedures by talking to these family members and others so that she could decide between three different procedures. She decided to go with the same approach I did and completed her surgery when she was on break. Then, what can I say? When my daughter-in-law's sisters and my daughter were all together to celebrate my son's birthday that year they had the opportunity to compare all their implants. Some families have many different things in common. For our family we seem to have had a steady stream of implants in our life. Me, my daughter, my daughter-in-law's sisters and even my step–daughter. We are taking the action that needs to be taken, we are choosing to be pro-active and decrease the risk of breast cancer. Strange life we lead some times. Yet, this follows my belief in controlling what you can.

I have already mentioned that the surgery went easily for me. Because life is full of changes I have now departed from the implant group. Last year, after more than seven years from my prophylactic surgeries, I developed an infection that housed itself in my implants and therefore they had to be removed. I had a great doctor again, and although I know I could get the implants again, that will probably not happen. My priority has to be treatment and certainly not any extra surgeries. I got the bras, the pads and no one knows the difference. I have also learned that when I am relaxing at the beach, I can forego everything.

So besides my daughter being positive, one of my sons tested negative and the other two still have to get tested. They know it and will do it, because they know I won't allow them not to.

Stability, Remission and Dancing with Ned

For almost ten years I traveled this journey stopping at all these stops along the way. After front line treatment I was told I was "Dancing with Ned". Not sure who or what Ned was, but I was thrilled to have the dance for twenty-one months. [NED is No Evidence of Disease] During that time, I wondered though, what was the difference between Ned and remission. Every other cancer seemed to call it remission, but for some reason we had Ned. But I liked Ned. He was a fine dancer. It took me awhile and then I realized nobody else understood what I was talking about except on my ovarian sites so I resorted to remission. Less complicated, and almost as exciting as Ned.

Then I used to wonder, how long before I reached the category of being a survivor. So many questions to ask myself over nine years. Not sure that word survivor ever worked for me. I still don't use it and only check it off when asked. I am more comfortable saying I am living with cancer. Maybe if it was gone I would feel I was surviving it, but I feel more like I am living it. Ok, that's what works for me. Everyone has to figure out what they are most comfortable with.

Stable... took me some time to get used to the fact "stable" was good on a scan. In the beginning I wanted to hear that the scan was clean. Doesn't seem to matter one bit what I would prefer. I can tell you now I would kill for stable. I realized a few years ago Ned has disappeared and so probably have the remissions. Now I set a new goal. Stable is it!

So, if I don't have remissions, can I have recurrences? Most likely not. After about four recurrences I started losing count. Plus, over the last three and a half years I have had no major breaks from treatment. I think, as I said before, I go back to my goal of stability.

I think I have already covered the topic, but it might help you to know how I lead my life. I work full time. I'm the director of a women's nonprofit. I have been on four clinical trials. At this juncture I can only do phase 1 trials. I keep looking. I have had four surgeries (five) if you count prophylactic mastectomy. Now I realize I have been on more than 8 different types of drugs. Again, really not counting unless I have to fill out someone's stupid forms. Oh, and there were also twenty-five treatments of targeted radiation. Easy to tolerate and gave me about nine months off until things percolated again. Only annoying thing was ice cream didn't really agree with me during radiation. I tend to have ice cream every night, but I managed to get through those times too. After all it was only five weeks.

The rest of my journey includes a wonderful and positive life. I play golf every week in summer, most frustrating game, but I find it my happy place. With my teal clothes, teal golf bag and my teal golf covers. I'm living the life. Living with my cancer. For now, I own it and schedule my treatments and trials around what is important to me.

Team Inspire is a tremendous resource and provides support for a multitude of cancers. Take advantage of the resources. Oh. and did I mention luck! I never for a minute underestimate the luck I have had through this journey. That and an amazing team of nurses and doctors running up and down the northeast corridor. With everything I have written and although there is much in this journey you can't control; you can be your own best advocate.

Trial and error

I have developed a habit when I get my ca125 results. If they start going up and there is a trend or larger than normal increase, the first thing I do is go to clinicaltrials.gov It is my go-to calming place. Strange, I know. For information purposes here, my ca125 is a pretty good indicator that something is percolating. If it goes up a few times in a row I start looking. As my doctor will say we don't treat the numbers we treat the scan. I know, I know, but so far, my theory has proven out for me. Everyone's numbers and different tumor markers mean and may show different things. When mine goes up I need to take some sort of action. I need to see what is out there. Having a plan enables me to feel a sense of control. Obviously not a huge amount of control, but enough to get me through the gaps. A few years ago, I posted a discussion on *Team Inspire* about rising ca125 and looking for something new out there. Someone responded and said, there is a great site for research clinicaltrials.gov, I said I know it well, it is on my speed dial.

To date, I have done four trials and almost got into a fifth (believe it or not I was eliminated because I didn't have enough cancer cells..., go figure).
First trial I tried to do in New York. But I had an insurance issue. They didn't take mine. Although drug company pays for the drugs, your doctor visits, scans etc. need to be covered by you or your insurance. This was for a vaccine trial when you had no disease. My husband and I decided that as long as my cancer wasn't active we should not make this major investment. We would wait until treatment was needed. But I continued my research and, go figure, I found the same trial at Hackensack Hospital, twenty minutes from my home. I didn't have to head in to NY and, most importantly, they took my insurance; keep trying and researching.

I was on the trial for fourteen months. I had the vaccine once a month. The day of my last vaccine (trial was ending) my scan showed the cancer was back. Never found out if I was getting a placebo or actual drug. That still annoys me! You know I tried to get that information.

What I did find out when the results were published was that the vaccine was shown not to be effective. Too bad, but research goes on, as do trials. Obviously not all will be effective, but they must continue.

My goal with trials was that I knew I could always try different chemo drugs that were approved, but I wouldn't always qualify for trials. Not exactly sure how and why I figured that out, but I did. I think the fact I also had BRCA mutation and it would exist potentially with my children I felt it important to be part of the process not just wait for solutions. I am not good waiting on sidelines.

So anytime a new treatment was necessary I preferred to do a trial. Not always available though. Since my home base doesn't do trials my doctor gave me the name of a doctor at NYU who was steeped in knowledge of ovarian trials. He also came up with ideas in between. With my BRCA status I really wanted to try a parp inhibitor trial if I could find one. We had a great dialogue (although my husband seems to feel I should let the doctor talk more) because I had done my homework.

Before my appointment I had located two places these trials were going on. U Penn and Dana Farber. I called both. U Penn was doing mid trial statistics and safety evaluations and wasn't enrolling, but Dana Farber was. They were amazing to work with and within 24 hours they sent me all the papers to read. I went to Boston and loved the staff. So, impressive. Turned out that my tumor was a little too small to enroll. Tumors need to show measurable disease which generally means it needs to be 2 cm. I was at 1.6. I left a little disappointed and then realized it was a good thing. Maybe I would get another six month break without treatment.

Just when we got really happy about that, within six weeks my ca125 doubled and then doubled again. Back in Boston pretty quickly and started the trial. Just an FYI it was the olaparib trial with cednarib. I was in the olaparib arm only which was fine since that was the drug I wanted. Only issues were my platelets (we will cover blood counts later). So, after three months the dosage was reduced in half, but I remained on the trial for nineteen months with 70% shrinkage before it started to grow.

I am a huge fan of the olaparib.
So what to do next....clinicaltrials.gov   again. Keep trying.

I had also been following what I considered my next plan that was a trial at U Penn where they did surgery and then collected your cancer cells to make a personalized vaccine. Sounded awesome to me. So, a few months later I headed to Penn for surgery. I was told there was little cancer left and therefore obviously not enough cancer cells to participate in the trial. Back on chemo a few months later to try and keep it at bay. There were no trials at this time out there to qualify for.

Fast forward another year. Since I continued my relationship with team at Dana, I was told there was another parp trial starting and I wasn't excluded. Yes! Got right up there and this time I had a different doctor, because it was on the research floor. No problem, great team, but after three months on this it wasn't working so off I came.

By then I was finding a trend with my research, I have been doing this a long time now; seven years. I was excluded from many things. So lesson #3, go to clinicaltrials.gov and find the things that I am watching (pd1, anti pd1 immunotherapy drugs, t-cells, vaccines, etc.) and read what the exclusions are first. Truly no point getting excited if I am excluded.
So here is the order: Search for type of cancer and type of drug, or type of cancer and city, or type of cancer and phase. The filters are great and help you figure out what is out there

Last trial I found out about was a phase 1 at Dana Farber. They called me the day it got final approval. Within three weeks I started the trial and within three more weeks I was off it. I felt great but my counts plummeted. My immune system tanked. I needed a platelet transfusion and shots. I was clearly not in a safety range for the trial. For information purposes here, one of the main priorities of phase 1 trials is safety. They explore combinations and dosages. I asked the doctor if three weeks was the fastest someone had come off a trial and she said no, but she did say I was the nicest. I'll go with that. I did find from my scan that the tumor shrunk a little. Who knows, my ca125 had spiked, so we have a little quandary but a good one. Smaller is smaller, less is less.

Final lessons learned for me... I have had so many treatments that I will never qualify for phase 2 or 3 trials. Just out of luck there. I can be that initial gerbil on the wheel for phase 1 trials. I am still good with that. I believe that for all cancers, progress will be made only if people step up and participate. Many drugs I have tried wouldn't be here if not for someone before me. So, it is important for me at any phase, for my children and for the future of those to come.

A cancer patient's life is always in flux. One scan, one lab report, one blood test can all send someone in a different direction. Recently I was stuck in the middle of trial crisis. My husband and I spent a week trying to decide whether I would participate in a trial at Memorial Sloan Kettering or a trial at U Penn. Ironically the goal of the trials was similar but the technology was different. We finally made the decision to do the Sloan trial because I would start within a two-week period and the U Penn trial for me wouldn't be able to begin until the end of November. Funny how decisions are made. Well to make matters interesting I spent ten days getting all the testing and dr appointments in to start the Sloan trial. Five days before starting I found out that there was a problem. My creatinine count (see chapter on counts) was too high. Ok, no problem, one option was to take IV fluids. Good news. It worked and brought it down. Following day I am getting ready for my scan and drinking their yummy raspberry drink. I get a call from the research nurse now saying that there is another problem and I may not need to do scan. Apparently, there is also a thing called creatinine clearance. Never heard of that before. Apparently, that number was too low. We came up with a plan but even I was a little discouraged. Here is life's irony.

When I got off the phone I saw I had a voice message from U Penn. Turns out they have a new opening if I am interested in the trial and could begin pretesting the following week. I called back and told them absolutely. Really hard to make these things up. So, Sloan did end up as an absolute no and Penn is the route of choice. In case anyone wonders this is a trial using my own T cells, modifying them over six weeks and then re-infusing them in my body. I am simply amazed at the new technologies.

I will be honest, traveling the path of trials is not always easy and clearly for my life there are lots of ways I get eliminated. But, I believe in them and will continue to pursue them as long as I can.

An important item to know is the new reality that if you are interested in a drug and can't seem to find a trial or qualify there is another option You can reach out directly to drug companies to try drug off trial. I have considered that route with immunotherapy drugs. I know I can get it, but I have also been made aware that right now it does not seem to be effective alone and is more effective when combined with a secondary drug. So, for me I wait. You can't always use these drugs twice so I shall watch and wait and maybe in the near future I will find a combo trial that is phase 1.

To count or not to count....

Half score - almost ten years ago....

It didn't take long for me to have issues with blood counts. I think I got one frontline treatment before we had to postpone treatment because of low platelet counts. So, my first protocol which was normally twenty-one days became every twenty-eight days. And so, it began.

When I began my IP cisplatin treatment, it was completed on a Friday. Felt miserable all weekend. Never thought about going to hospital. Waited until Monday and then called my oncologist. I didn't think much of it at the time, but by then my counts tanked, my pressure tanked, etc. Ended up in hospital for a week. Blood transfusions, platelet transfusion and the beginning of my counting skills. After that experience I also decided starting new treatments on Fridays was not the best idea. Since then I have avoided Friday starts. I am happier knowing I can reach my doctor the next day if there is a problem.

Over time, I tried to do what I could to counteract the plummeting counts. As I have said before being the best advocate for myself. I took aranesp (ouch: I think this is the most painful of the required shots) to help anemia and ward off blood transfusions (which became prevalent once numbers went below 9), the neulasta for the white cells (some people experience joint pain.... I was saved from that) so that became part of my regimen. I always ask my doctor whenever we start a new treatment if we should do neulasta and if it is warranted. If he says yes, then we always make sure it should be included. In terms of platelets, on the whole, all you can do is give them time to recover.

From frontline forth, my doctor began calling the different protocols, the protocol vs the 'Cathy Silverman' protocol. I work with it and stay completely on top of it.

It was a while after treatment and my twenty-one month dance with Ned that I did the carbo/taxol regimen again. From the start, I was on a twenty-eight day schedule. But this time I followed it with neulasta.

Managed through this pretty seamlessly. Maybe only one transfusion along the way. Unfortunately, Ned didn't feel like dancing too long.

I wanted to do doxil then. Go figure, the plant closed (who can make that up) and it wasn't available it he US. Alternate plan suggested: Radiation came and went, and then the Boston trial I mentioned. Let's see, back to the platelets. When on olaparib (lynparza) trial up in Boston at Dana Farber, I made it three months before platelets once again were getting to the no go range. So, fortunately for me the doctor was able to cut the dose from sixteen to eight pills a day and stick with the trial. That seemed to work and kept them under control. Managed for fourteen more months before progression returned. That was a pretty successful run in all ways with a majority of all my counts. The creatinine came close to being an issue, but I seemed to skate through. Not to mention I loved my olaparib.

I then had a very short period with doxil/avastin (soo ...not a friend of doxil.) I spent four months with what felt like thousands of glass shards in my throat before we decided no more. Definitely a mutual decision between me and my doctor. Ironically, counts were not an issue here. A few blisters, but those were manageable. And yes, I tried all the options out there for the mouth issues. Ironically, mouth issues yes, count issues no.

One thing about my doctor, he has shown some real flexibility with time. It used to be my platelets had to be over 100 for treatment. The mid 90s were a no go. Not so much anymore. Sometimes we even get down to 87ish. We work with all sorts of modifications that go along with the 'Cathy Silverman' protocol. Stay aware and continue to advocate!

Carbo/gemzar became the new plan in 2016. Doctor knew both could cause problems with counts so we went for lower dosages of both drugs. (I am the queen of lower dosages.). Always consider that option when discussing viable treatments with your doctor. So, about six weeks in and I am feeling great. It's my off week and I go to the Cancer Center for my normal lab work. It's 4:30 and it's after work and my plan is to go play some golf after. Feeling great as I said, just doing a finger prick. No big deal. I always wait for results. Then they tell me they had a problem with the read and they need to do it again, but with a vein. I suggest the port but they insist the vein. Ok, been going here a long time so I trust them, but I just try and save my veins. Then there seems to be more hubbub. Now they are looking at slides. I was then informed that my platelets were in a danger area "4" and the doctor needed to talk to me. (Feeling my golf game is not happening). I learned another new fact. When platelets get real low you also get lots of little red spots on legs called petechial. I was covered. Bruising I knew about. This was new. Feeling like I am knee deep in an on-line college course that just doesn't stop giving.

So, doctor says I need to have a platelet transfusion (been there done that) but I guess this one was more disconcerting. It's now 5:00 PM. Looking like Ugh, I might be headed to emergency room because of time, cross check blood, etc. I sweetly ask if there is any chance they could get it done while I was still in the infusion center. Unlikely I'm told but will check with supervisor. Doctor calls over and supervisor says we will take care of it for Cathy, just send her right here. (Only across hall so easily done.) Major lesson, love your nurses and be nice, they are one of your best advocates, they do what they do for a reason. They are the best. They stayed late and so did the doctor. Got it done but once again I got to see my doctor's artwork. He drew many pictures and scenarios about what could have caused this. What we were hoping for and what we were not. It went the right away for me and by the end of the night my platelets bumped up 45 points. I learned something else that night. After seven years I found out my doctor's specialty was hematology. Who knew?

Not a surprise, no golf that day, but I did go out on the weekend. And, as you can imagine no more carbo/gemzar. Gemzar alone was easy on my counts. I guess I should say easier. We still watched dosing though. Unfortunately, it stopped working after only a few months. So, I needed a combo. Next up or back, cisplatin/gemzar. My doctor once told me I would never again be on cisplatin. I was good with that, though. As you can already imagine the dose was very low, I mean very low dose. Still watched the counts and the doctor still modified the dose when platelets went down. But the main thing was we managed about six months (again, I was feeling great) until it was clear that numbers and here I mean ca125 was not going well. I   started researching a new plan. I spoke and traveled to other members of team to see what trials might be around for me, but nada. So, we decided to try taxol; three weeks on and one week off.

Here comes one of the funniest stories of my journey. So again, I started with low dose taxol so the doctor can try and get my numbers steady. I think the dose was 45 ml (don't ask me what 45 exactly is), but ok I get it. So, the following week, platelets are up from previous week so I ask (please always ask, you are your best advocate) what dose am I getting. He says 45 again. I said, but my numbers are better, can't we go higher? He asks, would 60 make me happy? I say yes.

Fast forward to the following week, I am sitting in the infusion waiting area, counts are done but I haven't seen them yet and my phone rings. It is a Cancer Center number. I answer and it is my nurse (my doctor's nurse). She is laughing. I ask what is so funny. I just picked up the phone. She tells me she has never made a call like this. Ok, what is it? She says my doctor told her to call me and ask me what dose I want. I say that means that numbers are even better, right, she says yes. I say I can go up to 75 right, she says yes. I say let's do it then! I still find this pretty funny myself. I love that he listens to me, knows me and lets me be my best advocate.

After this treatment, I got a call that the next trial in Boston was approved and I had a spot. As I previously mentioned I lasted three weeks because my counts all completely crashed. Back at my home base we decided to steer the course back to taxol.

Funny story continues. I'm there for my first treatment again. Low and behold, my platelets are at 205. I don't think they have ever been at 205. I guess that is what being off treatment for three weeks does. It's just been a long time since I had that type of break. Not seeing the doctor that day because I knew he was at his own doctor's appointment; very informed am I. So, I go back to treatment room. I am not sure who put order in that day since my nurse was also on her honeymoon. I ask my infusion nurse my typical question. "What is the dose? " today? She says 60. I say not happening. You have to reach out to Doctor G and increase it to 75. My platelets are 205 and we are so not doing only 60. She laughs, says she will call and runs to pharmacy to stop them from getting drugs ready. Five minutes later she comes in and says 75, all good. Again... gotta advocate.

Last story on counts, sat with the doctor going over previous trial experience and plans for moving forward and he says you didn't cover everything. I ask what did I miss? He says I didn't tell him what dose am I having that day. I asked, is this the highest dose that is used with taxol. He said no. I asked then, will I be able to go higher than 75. He also says no. He explains that he has to keep things at a certain level so we don't have bone marrow damage. I'm ok then, 75 it is. I know when to advocate and I also know when to trust. Know that you have the best team of doctors looking out for you. Survival depends upon it.

I am adding some thoughts about a month after I wrote this section. I have a funny anecdote to add to this story. I am resolved that 75 is the maximum dose I can receive of Taxol.   All of a sudden one day, as is my usual question before we start treatment, what is the dose? My nurse says 80.   Now I was really surprised. No complaint of course, just surprised. So, I see my doctor a few hours later and of course I had to question how we were higher than 75? He had told me that was my limit. He explained that it is a formula and is based upon my weight that day (I guess I had a large dinner the night before or maybe a large lunch), my weight was up about two or three pounds, so the formula increased to 80. I then clarified, so if I want to remain two or three pounds heavier than I currently am I can stay at 80. He said probably. I gave it some thought and said nah, I don't think so. I like my weight where it is. Only going from 75-80 was not enough motivation to change my vanity.

Scanning Around

What type; Where to go; how often; ….. Although I know that many doctors use CT scans, there are some who do Pet scans or even MRIs. I pretty much have been on the CT scan circuit. Once in a while a Pet scan has been used to clarify a CT scan, but it's been at least six years since that happened to me.

I included a where to go here question because of my experience. For many years I did my scan at a facility that was outside of the hospital but affiliated with it. Every time I had a scan…. I was asked the same thing by someone from the insurance company. "Do you know you could do your scan somewhere else locally and you would have a lower co-pay?" My answer was always the same, yes but this is where I want it done. My rationale was easy…. They do the scan and it gets uploaded right in to the computer and my doctor has easy access to it. Then one day I had an issue with my creatinine level in terms of the contrast. So, they wouldn't do it at the Ambulatory Center. Then I needed it to be done at the hospital so they could give me IV fluids first. No big deal, but I did find it interesting that they had a different protocol for how much and when to drink the yummy barium. They pretty much required not one, but two bottles to drink. (By the way my drink of choice has always been the banana flavor.) Again, got a call from insurance company who also asked the same question…. "do you know you could do your scan locally somewhere else?" Yes, same answer and rationale.

It was about four years ago that I was going over some scan bills and the amount of co-pay and it seemed like I was really paying a lot. I decided to do some research. I contacted my insurance company (the one that always called) and asked specific questions regarding the costs. What the co-pay was at the Ambulatory Center, the hospital and a radiology group (which they had mentioned to me) located about 5 minutes from my home. Wow, what a difference. I was actually paying about $300 more per scan by doing it at the hospital. Since at that juncture in time I was doing about four per year (sometimes even more when I was on a clinical trial) that came out to more than $1200 out of my pocket per year. Let alone the number of years.

No surprise here, I made a change. I'd rather save my money for something I may need treatment related down the road. I make the system work easily for me. And ironically when I am doing trials this system actually works better. I stay right after my scan until they burn the disc and then I overnight it to the Cancer Center where I am headed or keep an extra one with me when I might be doing my travels.

Another advantage this change has had was that it is a smaller facility and I have gotten to the know the techs better. One day at my visit, it was later than normal and I was talking to my techs and she was surprised I was that late. I told her it was the earliest I could get. She then told me if I ever had a problem just call and speak to her. She would quietly move me earlier on the schedule. She knows I come appropriately dressed and I am really quick so she was so happy to do it. And to be honest I did need her to do it at least once for me. Remember what I said earlier. So many people in this medical business are committed to making our lives easier. Be nice to everyone and treat them with respect. They each care for us in their own ways. Now in terms of why I like to go early. There are two reasons, 1) I go to work right afterwards and 2) most importantly I can usually get the report from scan faxed to me by the end of the day. Huge!!! I really like seeing the report right away.

Now, how often to have the scan. That too varies where someone is on treatment. If you are in remission or NED, then you probably go every three months or six months or once a year depending how long you have gone. If you are in treatment completely different. Insurance wise unless you are on a trial, they generally don't like to approve a scan in less than 90 days. They will under certain circumstances, but they don't like to.

Since I have been on steady treatment for a while now, my scheduling really varies. Years ago, I might have thought I would go every month. But that doesn't happen so much anymore. If my ca125 is remaining "fairly" stable, then I just keep up with treatment. On the other hand, if it starts jumping up and up you can be sure I set that scan up quickly.

23

To quote my doctor, we don't treat a ca125; we treat what is on the scan. I would say in the last two years I went nine months without a scan because things were stable. This year I did January, April (May again because of a HUGE spike and I was on a trial) then August. Here is where you work things out with your doctor. The one thing I truly regret is that when I had my surgery three years ago, we didn't do a scan afterwards. I know the doctor got everything visible and my ca125 was back to the normal range, but it just would have been nice to see a clean scan. Not particularly relevant to anyone but me, but it would have been nice. Figured I didn't need to put the extra contrast in my body either.

To Operate or Not to Operate

What I really hate is when I am in a medical office and I have to fill out the section related to previous surgeries. It really brings out the dread in me.

The list has grown over the years and honestly my theory has changed. During my first three years I had three abdominal/pelvic surgeries. My original two surgeries in the first three months, then my prophylactic mastectomy and then another one for my first recurrence. I used to joke that I could use Velcro. My cancer has been in the same spot each time. It apparently has located itself there for the duration. People would ask me if I was going to have surgery again down the road. I explain that I didn't think too many surgeries were a good idea. That was my interpretation at the time without much to back it up. All things do change though.

Three years ago, I had my last surgery. That was in order to qualify for a trial with a personal vaccine. Good news, I didn't have enough cancer cells. Better news was we got everything cleaned out again. Since that time and a variety of treatments I started thinking that what I'd really like is to try another surgery and clean it out again. If I could do this every few years, it would seem to make great sense to me. But alas, that would be too easy.

In researching what I could do again, I brought up this possibility when I needed a change in treatment at the beginning of the year. Unfortunately for me I have been given pretty clear no's by two of the doctors on my team. It seems that although my tumor is only in one spot, as it has slightly grown, it has encroached in an area that would make future surgery much more damaging. C'est la vie. I guess surgery will be put on the back burner until I don't have so many real options out there. But I will always know that it exists as a last resort when other things are failing. It's just hard when you simply want it gone.

Team Sports and How to Recruit

When I started this journey, I had three doctors. My gynecologist, my gynecological oncologist and my oncologist. I love and respect each one of them. I live thirty minutes outside of New York City, but I knew I was getting top notch treatment. I didn't go for second opinions but knew I could if needed. What I did know was that my center did not do trials. So, began the formation of my team.

When I coached soccer (which I did for years) or drove my kids to practice to different club teams, it was always important to have the right players and right personnel. So, as I began my education for trials, so began the development of my team. It wasn't an active search, it was in some ways trial and error. My oncologist first recommended a doctor at NYU. He was great leading us in directions and coming up with ideas. I guess he was the first member.

But major changes did occur when I first visited Dana Farber. When I met the doctor there she blew me away from the first minute. Her knowledge of my particular cancer and everything I had done and the trial she was doing were a perfect match. I doubt she even knows how excited I was when I met her. The nineteen months of that trial only cemented it for me. She and her nurse are always my first go to people when Dr. G and I know there are changes imminent. Ironically it was the first major expansion of my team because at my hospital it is a general practice with some specialties, so she was my first added star in my specialty. She gives us ideas and Dr. G helps me evaluate the right path.

Once that ended I went to Philadelphia pursuing my next trial. In order to qualify I needed to do surgery at U Penn. The doctor running the trial became the next member of my team. He was the researcher, oncologist and surgeon. Unfortunately, that trial didn't pan out, but the surgery was hugely successful.

At different points in my journey I came across trials that interested me at Sloan Kettering in NY. My beginning experiences were not great. I wanted simple answers about open trials and they wanted all my pages and pages of records before they would comment. Then they still wouldn't comment. I had to come in. I met with one doctor there who was very very nice, but he didn't set my heart aflame. The competition to get on my team started to get harder.

When you get knocked down, you get back up and so a year later when I wanted to go back to Sloan, I switched doctors. In terms of advocating, this is your team and you get to make the decisions and call the plays. It took two weeks for me to get approval to change doctors at the same hospital, but I was determined and it happened. Aside from the fact he looked like he was twelve, he impressed me immediately. There were no trials for me there so I told him which ones I was considering in Boston. Without a seconds delay he said exactly which one I should do and why. That became my decision and aside from the fact I got beat out by someone on the waiting list it would have been great.

And that leads to who is currently the last member of the team until something else changes. The last two trials that I ended up doing at Dana Farber were each with a different doctor. One who specializes in research not just ovarian. She too has been amazing. These are my go-to peeps. My team can't always be measured in wins and losses but is considered successful when I experience every wedding, new grandchild and family event.

I am very fortunate to live in the northeast corridor. I even have children near NIH in Maryland but haven't used that as a resource yet. I am sure this too will happen. Wherever you are, you must be aware of your resources. If you don't know them, ask. If you need and have the ability to travel be aware of that as well. Whatever helps with this fight stay on it. YOU are important.

Your team may be a team of one or a team of many. There are other people who are involved with team sports. They support your major players even though your oncologists and or surgeons may be up there at the top. There are also a multitude of specialists that may be brought in as needed. Whether it is a gastro doctor, an infectious disease doctor, a urologist, a nephrologist (didn't remember I had one

27

previously until I needed one again), or the multitude of other specialties that exist out there but are there to help you any way they can. It is important to always know that if you need some additional substitutions there are other people out there. You are too important to limit yourself if need arises.

Caregivers: The Team's Designated Hitter

This is a topic that is a little unique for me to include here. It is not an experience that I have personally had. It is not an experience that I have personally had. I have been the recipient of care. I have not been dealt the hand of someone who has been thrown full force into caring for someone with cancer and all of the issues and implications that come with it. What I can relate to is how important it is to us all. The love and support that comes through on so many different levels. The fears, the emotions, the highs the lows, the doctors' appointments, the tests, the whole and entire change of life once a diagnosis and treatment become reality. On-going treatment change the lives of caregivers forever.
All I can say is that I am grateful for the people in my life that I know are there every day

Is There Anything Scarier than Drug Commercials?

Have you ever watched a commercial on TV for a drug and by the time they finished listing the side effects you wondered why anyone could possibly want to take it? You could experience, nausea, vomiting, weight gain, weight loss, constipation, diarrhea, back pain, leg pain, head pain etc., etc. It sounds like the drug could kill you.

Not unlike the experience with chemo. Clearly, we are putting poisons and toxins in our bodies. For those who it helps that go into remission, it seems like a good bet. For those who remain on constant treatment it enables us to live.

Yet, sometimes it seems that the side effects can throw you over the edge. Personally, I have to admit that I have been pretty fortunate and lucky. I had one situation when I was on frontline treatment and started losing my hair. That is a perfectly normal symptom and we all know when going on certain drugs that will be the case. But no one I spoke with had ever heard about what I experienced. In the first two weeks of treatment. I developed scabs all over my head. I felt like a porcupine. I had about 200 scabs and felt sharp pains all over my head. Could barely place my head on a pillow. Strange. Fortunately, my husband found an article written by oncology nurses with some photos and descriptions. Sure, enough it was similar to what I had, but mine was unbelievably worse. I was put on an antibiotic I never heard of and it worked immediately. Now that it is a little simplification, but let me explain. The doctor gave me a few samples. But when I went to the pharmacy they had a hard time getting the approval. They gave me the generic but explained that there might be some side effects. Seriously. The samples had been easy. The pharmacy ones made me nauseous. So, I handled all the chemo without being nauseous but the idiotic antibiotic put me over the edge. Thank goodness, I called the doctor back and got more samples. They did the trick without any other issues. Remember always advocate for yourself. Afterwards I then shared the photos and article with my doctor and the nurses in the infusion center. I have felt compelled from the beginning that if I learned information that was not commonly known (which clearly was the case here) it was important to share it where I could. I keep all sorts of articles in my files so at a moment's notice I can simply spread the wealth of knowledge I have accumulated.

On frontline and the second time with carbo/taxol I didn't have one day of nausea. That is one of the most common side effects from so many chemos. My diet wasn't great. I did have the metallic taste, but worked my way through a few months of pizza and sometimes French fries. Oh, and orange drink from McDonalds. Strange, right? Anyway, there has to be a silver lining. The pizza slice had a beginning middle and end so I pushed myself to finish a slice. I lost about fifteen pounds, but I was kind of a fan of that. I know so many people struggle with so much more and there is no question there are side effects that can kill someone. But as we all know without the treatment the alternative sucks! So, on we go and hope for the best.

Truly the worst issue I have dealt with is the mouth sores from the doxil. I did it, and I admit for me it was life altering until we cut the treatment short. I only managed four cycles. Couldn't talk, couldn't eat, felt like I had thousands of glass shards in my mouth. Periodically a little Percocet got me through a day. Never liked to take it, but occasionally I had to manage it. All in all, not so much fun! Yet, I would do it again in a heartbeat if that was my option. Ironically once off the doxil I had a few months with avastin only. Then I went to the dentist. Within two days the mouth issues were back. Not awful and fairly manageable. But I will admit it took me longer than normal to step back into my dentist's office.

I have a hunch (not to mention three different treatments since then) that I now have a predisposition for mouth issues. When you read the side effects of a drug and it says less than 10% of the people experience mouth issues. I have become one of them. Even on drugs I had pre doxil, when I have them now I have the issues. I am working it though. It is not the glass shards again which helps. It is more like my mouth getting prickly. I watch the foods with acids and alcohol. Oh, and talking. I talk a lot at work and at home and on the golf course and in general. Sometimes it is the talking alone that can set things in motion but not much I can do about that. It is not real pain I experience so I can tolerate the prickliness.

If I have treatment on a Tuesday, I am good until sometime Thursday. It will flare after two or three days. Only recently I calculated I might be able to sneak in bruschetta on a cracker on Wednesday night since it is going to flare up Thursday regardless of what I do Wednesday. Sometimes Sunday or Monday nights before treatment, Tuesdays are ok as well. I don't overdo it though. Haven't tried to go for a full order of veal parmigiana either. Since treatment is three weeks on and one week off, I can really splurge on my off week. Pizza…. I so miss pizza and tomato sauce. Recently on my off week at the beach I went for Italian food (really excellent in NJ). I think I had three slices of pizza, then I shared a pasta with vodka sauce and some with plain spaghetti sauce etc. It was so so good.

I have heard so many side effects and issues that people experience. I wish I could help people with other things and with hints to get through some of these side effects but it is hard to help when I haven't experienced them. Please don't forget to have discussions with your doctor and the infusion nurses. There may be some ways to minimize side effects. Not completely and not always or not at all. I don't want to make a prediction or promise. Potentially you can spread out the time between treatments, or lower the dosages. Again, be your own best advocate and ask the questions. If you recall in a previous section I thought I would never be on cisplastin again. But I was and I handled it perfectly. We utilized a much, much smaller dose and a lot of hydration. Made it through six months. So again…. Advocate.

Emergency rooms or trauma – are they the same?

Let me start with the positives here. Emergency Rooms are necessary and the staff who work there are dedicated personnel and only want to help. They are there when your Cancer Centers are closed and you really need emergency services. I am grateful for that.

Having said that, they are not always easy. They can be amazingly crowded which leads to long wait times and not always good times. But you have no choice when the need arises. Advice here, do it nicely, but make sure you are your own best advocate. You can be nice but strong at the same time.

About a year ago I thought I was doing both, but in hindsight even I, and that surprises me, didn't do enough. I was at the Cancer Center with a high fever with no reason we could identify. I needed to be admitted. It was the end of the day and there were no open rooms. So, therefore the emergency room was where I was headed. My nurse even walked us over because she wanted to move it along. There was a long line to check in and I finally told her to head back upstairs, I could take care of it. After all, my doctor had also already called over since I was being admitted. So, I finally got to the receptionist and explained that it was not a good idea for me to be in the waiting room with a lot of people. She explained that I would be seen by the triage nurse and they would take care of that. I also asked for a mask in the meantime. There were barely any seats available and probably about fifty people waiting. Not a good sign. So, I waited to be called by the triage nurse. Thirty minutes, an hour, an hour and a half. Not so happy right now. A lovely hospital administrator came down and explained the shortage of rooms and the backlog of people and was truly apologetic. She also brought a large cart of drinks and a variety of snacks which were appreciated. After she finished speaking I asked if we could talk to her. I explained that I was running a high fever, had been sent down by my doctor in the Cancer Center and that I really needed to be out of waiting area. I told her I still had not been called by triage and it was almost 2 hours. She told me she would be right back. After a few minutes, she had the triage nurse call us. She took my temp and with over 103 degrees, she said you shouldn't be out here. Duh! Right away they at least took me to the inside triage area away from the waiting room. I still had to wait a short time but they definitely moved me up in front of about 30 people. Live and learn. I said all the right things, but should not have let it go that long.

I haven't been to the emergency room that often, but go figure, ended up there a few weeks later with another fever. This time not so crowded but I did go over right away to the triage desk and explained my situation. I did not wait until I was called. They couldn't have been nicer and moved me out of waiting room right away. The staff was great, but the wait some time can be difficult. Know when you really need to act and just be nice about it.

Although neither of these er visits were related to treatment, I made a decision anyway. I try and set up my treatments midweek if possible so that it gives me the ability to seek assistance with my own doctor and the Cancer Center rather than it be a weekend and a trip to the Emergency Room.

Home is Where The Heart Is

Perspective is an interesting concept. I think there are those that would think I am a wee bit nuts when I say I feel like I am home when I am at my Cancer Center. In some ways, you get what you give. I am always, and I mean always, happy to see everyone there. After all this time, they know me pretty well. They really are all part of my life and they do what they can to make my life easier and I know they care. They know when I have my hair cut, when I wear a fun outfit for treatment or probably when it's simply the end of a long work day. We talk about children, weddings, life events and obviously cancer. We talk, we laugh and sometimes we even cry. That is what you do with family and friends.

I was in the elevator one day with another cancer patient and as we were getting off I mentioned something about what a great place this was and how happy I was to be there. I think she thought I was crazy. I then explained my thoughts and how I feel fortunate to be in such a great place with such wonderful people. Besides I explained…. the alternative sucks!!

Everyone has different experiences though. I have been to five other hospitals during this journey of mine. My home base at RWJ Barnabas and my trial base at Dana Farber truly exemplify these experiences. This is not at all a statement about the other hospitals and staffs I have utilized, it is simply that I have, in fact, developed long-term and longstanding relationships in both of these places. I do recommend though, if you do not feel comfortable that you are in the best place that you could be, look at your options. It's like the old TV show, Cheers. It's nice to be in a place where everyone (maybe not everyone…) knows your name.

Luck and/or Faith

I don't want to be ungrateful or cynical when I say that often people tell me how inspirational I am or they talk about how I handle my situation. I work with hundreds of women in my community so there are many people who know my story. I wish I could tell you that I have done something to be inspirational. But that really isn't the case. I admit I am the type of person who looks at my cup as half full. That hasn't changed. I, like millions of others, have been dealt this hand that no one wants to play; the club no one asks to join. But how we approach it is very individual and based upon a multitude of circumstances.

Lots of things go into that approach. Believe me, I am not looking for accolades. In its simplicity, I want to live. I want to watch my family grow and participate in all of life's celebrations. I work diligently to give myself the best advantages I can by being as knowledgeable as I can. When hearing myself talked about in this manner, I truly try and explain certain things about my situation. I am not the only one who advocates, creates a good team or stays on top of my situation. But so far, while I have done all those things, I never negate the fact I consider myself very, very lucky. I know that seems like a strange statement from someone dealing with cancer for almost ten years. But I am here to write these words. I have lost many friends to cancer. Many of them were activists as well. They educated themselves, they did clinical trials, they traveled across the world to simply be able to live. They wanted to watch their families grow as well. We talked on discussion boards, went for dinner in cities far away from home; And yet I survive and, simply put, they did not. Their memory reminds me that I have been lucky and maybe even blessed.

Some people say it is my attitude that helps. I certainly believe it doesn't hurt, but again, nothing is ever so simple. For those throwing up daily from chemo it is hard to feel like you can get out of bed and pull yourself out of some sort of depression. When your bones ache and you spend hours in the bathroom it is not always easy to see that full cup. I am not saying that there aren't people who see the cup empty. I am guessing they have a harder time. But don't judge, just try and be supportive.

Since I have been trying to find the humor here while I put these words on paper, you should know, for me, in all this time I can only remember throwing up twice. The first was from an antibiotic I was taking for the side effect I had with head issues and we were on the way home from my picking my dress for my son's wedding. We had to pull the car over and that was that. The one that is most memorable (and again I am so fortunate that my chemo treatments haven't revolved around being sick) was in the middle of the train station in Boston and not near a garbage can or a bathroom. I was on a clinical trial and my flight was canceled because of bad weather and so I was going to take the train home. In the middle of the train station, that was it. I can actually look back on that evening and still find some humor in it. That was my last day on that trial. It wasn't working. And we decided after 3 months it was time to move on. I can find the humor much more readily now, but when I was in the middle of the train station…. Probably not so much.

Treatment can be devastating due to the side effects. I have been lucky enough that for all but four months of my treatments my side effects have been "manageable". Those four months, as I said, the mouth sores made my quality of life a little bit of hell. OK, a lot of hell. But you know what, I would do it all over again if I need to. If doxil would be an option I needed to repeat… then I would say bring it on. Hence, I consider myself lucky. How you feel and how you can function impacts your attitude and your life.

Recently, I got to relook at my luck as well as my perspective. I realized that along with what I determined was luck, was also the fact that in some ways with the manageable side effects that I experienced, up until now I could easily deal with side effects. Yet, in actuality I really didn't have to deal with what I consider complications. It does give perspective. As previously discussed my treatment options become less as my resistance to chemo increases and my options for trials is diminished. For me this means I have to actually start prioritizing treatment and decisions over my life and work. Have to say I don't like it at all. But, tumor is growing and creating blockages which must be dealt with. Had a grim day in evaluating options but I gave myself a day to let it sink in. Then I reached back up and did my research and continued meeting with my team. And the only way I function when evaluating complications is to choose living. So, if this means life changing treatments or surgery, so be it. I can adjust to anything as long as I can be around to live life.

I include faith in the title of this chapter because I know that for many people faith gets them through their days. Just as I have a positive attitude and consider myself lucky I know that faith is what helps others go through their journeys. As far as I am concerned whatever can help is the direction you take.

Advocate…. Knowledge is power

I have mentioned advocating for yourself throughout this story. I can't overstate this. Your life depends on it. No one but you have a stronger interest in surviving cancer. No doctor should be put off by your questions. And if they are, you need to get a new doctor. My doctor knew in the beginning I always came prepared with a list of questions. I started with a pad of paper and lists. Then I got more technological and my questions were on my phone or iPad. This also became more effective because I always have my phone with me so if I think of something at work or out and about I can type it out and have it for my next visit, I don't have to remember until I have paper and pen.

I have always, always believed that knowledge is power. Own the power. How to educate yourself now and by that, I mean in 2017. When I was first diagnosed I was told to be careful what I read on the internet. That is true. But there are amazing support systems and educational opportunities to learn about and to search for on the internet. I have learned a tremendous amount on these sites and by participating on discussion threads. You can ask questions and hear a multitude of responses from people going through the same treatment regimens. You can hear about successes and failures. You can learn about side effects and sometimes things you can do to minimize them. Not every community offers on-site support groups. These internet sites can provide support systems for you and or family members if you choose. We all have questions and we all have information we can share.

Team Inspire is a site that has groups for different cancers. I am not sure about everything that is included, but it is something to pass on to those in need. They provide like-minded cancer communities. Look and see what is offered for you. They are now my home base especially because two of the other ones which existed nine years ago have shut down. I get tremendous information from this site and have formed some incredible long-term Internet relationships and sadly lost too many.

Force is a website for the BRCA mutation. If you have this in your family, they are beyond amazing. Whether you have been tested or not, every piece of information you may need can be located there. They offer educational webinars, discussion threads, listings of clinical trials for breast and ovarian, surgery information and many more items for both men and women. Although breast and ovarian are the most common, if you carry the gene you have more of a pre-disposition to other cancers as well. Please check it out if anyone you know is BRCA positive or if breast or ovarian cancer run in someone's family; so they can determine if they should be tested.

Officially, become an advocate. Attend a conference, go to Washington DC, involve yourself with a local or national organization for your cancer. This is the one area that I have not taken the jump in yet. I go to DC for my job every few years and unfortunately one of the conferences for Ovarian Cancer is always in July. I'm just not prepared to give up a beach weekend at the Jersey Shore for a conference. I do send letters on line, even to the FDA. Find what works for you. We all can decide what we are comfortable with and what we have the energy or priority to do.

Just to reiterate…. Don't stay in the dark. Learn and question and make sure you get the best care and best chances you can. We only have this one life to live.

Recently I have been in touch with someone with a family member being diagnosed with cancer. They were waiting for biopsy and scan results.

The questions that I sent to her are listed in the Appendix. These are questions which cross over all cancer lines. The fact that is was 1:30 AM was irrelevant.

The Changing World We Live in

Chemo, radiation and surgery were all the rage when I first began the journey.

Who ever heard of immunotherapy? Opdivo, keytruda.... PD1; Anti Pd1 just to mention a few; Chk 1, Parps etc....

Four years ago when I did my parp inhibitor trial they were in beginning stages and nothing had been presented to the FDA. Who could have imagined that in this same time period now there are three different parp inhibitor drugs that have received some sort of approval by the FDA.

With so many cancers and so many drugs and trials there are so many things in flux. But this is a good thing. Drugs we never heard of a few years ago have become a part of different cancer treatments and varying protocols. Once a drug gets approved for one cancer, trials begin for other cancers. It is good for the drug companies and of course for us, the patients. Either way, all good.

T-cell trials; harvesting cancer cells and creating personalized vaccines for treatment; who could have imagined this when I began.

Every day I get my Google Alert for ovarian cancer. (An alert can be set up for all/any cancers and it is a way to stay informed and educated once again.) I read about any new trials or achievements that are related to "my" cancer. Then I send it to myself so I have it when it might come in handy or if I want to ask my doctor about it. I guarantee that every day I read articles about something I have never heard of before. It gives me such hope. I can remember the time sitting in Dr. G's office for my first appointment when he told us the goal was to treat this as a chronic disease. It seemed so far-fetched at the time. I wanted to be cured. Who doesn't? But it didn't take long to take that philosophy to heart. (Especially since I really only had 1 significant remission). We truly are treating it as a chronic disease. We take the drugs/trials to beat it down and when it stops working we regroup, come up with a new plan and start all over.

But the possibilities give me hope. We are learning about genomes, new tests for specific cells (not my expertise here) instances where a treatment not approved for your cancer can be approved because your tumor has something that exists for another cancer thereby allowing you to get approved for the drug. I think that was a long run on sentence but I am trying to make a point and I really am lacking the specific knowledge and training on this one

Vice President Biden began the moonshot program: Stand up to Cancer brought together experts doing research in every field. What else exists but for us to keep fighting and keep hoping. If we hang out long enough the development of new drugs and new protocols will enable us to keep living just a little bit longer. I am excited, but don't think I am not realistic. I no longer worry about cures. I am not even talking about remissions for me anymore. (Though it would be great.) I am simply talking about survival and living with the disease.

I feel compelled here to also add a thank you. I am not trying to thank myself here. To those who have put themselves out and done clinical trials (and the reason I feel so strongly about participating in them), is because each and every person and each and every trial enables the future to be brighter.

Finding your happy place

I have definitely learned to appreciate many things and to also let go of the small stuff (most of the time). I recommend strongly that everyone really think about what makes you happy. You'd be surprised what you come up with. I think the process itself will bring you some joy. I know that it did it for me.

Simple things bring a smile to my face. My ringtones. Phones ring all the time. Why not make it something that makes you happy? At first it was Kelly Clarkson's "Stronger". I saw a video which was made in a Cancer Center with a patient and the nurses. What is happy? A song, a smile, a laugh. This video and then the song did all three. Loved hearing it on the radio, but even more every time my phone rang.

After a while I think my family was getting tired of it though. That wouldn't have bothered me but at the same time on the Ellen DeGeneres show there was a teenage girl who had just finished treatment for cancer. She had been in her school's talent show and sang Rachel Platt's "The Fight Song". That day Ellen surprised the girl. Rachel Platt was there and they sang it together. Changed my ring tone that day. A little thing but it makes me happy whenever my phone rings.

You already know golf is one of my happy places. I have become obsessed, even though it is the most frustrating game. Yet a few hours on the course with my husband and friends are a wonderful way to spend an afternoon. Especially if I get more good shots than bad.

An absolutely necessity and one of my favorite times of the week is playing mah jong. Playing with my friends is wonderful, but when they can't all make it, I rarely miss the opportunity to put a game together with my cadre of subs.

Work, did I say I love my job? It makes me happy. I am passionate about the work I do and about the people I spend my every day with. My organization works to improve lives of women, children and families. Obviously it takes the better part of my week but it's the best place to be and the best job to do.

Traveling also makes me happy. From seeing new sights to visiting an island or hanging out at our beach house. I love the down time. I need the relaxation. I have to prioritize where I want to go and what I want to do. I visited a special resort last winter and I truly found a happy place. Beautiful beaches, a little piece of paradise, great massage and wonderful friends. Oh, and did I mention a banana daiquiri or two. Definitely happy. Do something special for yourself.

Reading makes me happy. I have to admit, I intersperse a few serious novels in my selections, but I really stick with romance novels and sometimes some that are a little trashy. I read some mysteries as well. I just can't deal with the too too serious always. Ironically it's amazing how many people in these books are dealing with cancer. Life, is life and books can't always be a complete escape. Yet, it really makes me happy. Whether it is at night before I go to sleep, on my porch at the beach or when I am away on a vacation.

Here's a surprise, Facebook. Connecting with family and friends. Being able to share a piece of those who mean something and some who may be on the fringe, but none the less a way to stay in touch. I love to see the photos of celebrations and what is happening to people I care about. Although my children sometimes used to think I was stalking a little, too bad. It brings me to my happy place.

Very important to me and certainly something I rarely miss in a day is chocolate. I have been a chocoholic as long as I can remember. I have a special weakness for dark chocolate and I always keep some of the good stuff in my desk at my office. I guess here I can mention that I pretty much also have some type of chocolate ice cream every night. We may not have much food in our refrigerator, but the freezer must have chocolate ice cream. Having said this, I think this is the appropriate place for what I thought was a funny chocolate cancer story.

I had just had a not so enjoyable sandwich while at Sloan waiting for my appointment for IV fluids. I finally decided I needed chocolate so I went over to the receptionist and asked where I might be able to find some. (They generally have saltines and graham crackers in every waiting room.) I was told to go to the 11th floor. I go over to the elevator and a woman in a scarf asks me if I am a cancer patient. I replied yes and then she proceeded to tell me that I should not have any chocolate. She said that sugar is very, very bad for cancer. I thought very quickly but responded to her and explained that I have been on this cancer journey for almost ten years and no one takes away my chocolate…. But thanks for caring. I thought I handled it nicely, which was pretty good since it had already been a long day and I really really needed my chocolate.

I guess shopping should also be mentioned. I love wearing something new right after I buy it. I don't do so much shopping in stores but when I do, it is more fun than on-line. I have also learned that I can justify some extra shopping when I need some retail therapy. It becomes imperative when ca125 goes up or a scan shows growth. Got to keep feeling good.

This one may also seem a little strange. I am happy that I spend treatment time with the most amazing professionals and staff. From those who do registration
to the lab techs, nurses assistants and doctors. We talk, we laugh. Their caring is evident in everything they do. The relationships that have been created defy
description. We really care and love each other. During every visit spent together they give a part of their hearts. They work in a field with so many highs and devastating lows and they care so much. They make me incredibly happy.

And a project at the hospital, Comfort Project 360: what happiness they are bringing to us all at the Cancer Center. They bought soft furry robes for radiation, appointments and doctor visits. They have taken tired looking waiting areas and hallways and transformed them to warm, cheery comfortable rooms for what are sometimes long waiting times with the frightening aspects of cancer treatment.

Soon each infusion room will be remade as well. All new patients will see a smiling face and get a warm comfy blanket and a great hat. And of course, one of my favorites, the Comfort Cart. There is the food I depend on to get me through the treatment. It is the best comfort food. Candy, chocolate, chips and nuts (nourishing things as well) and I could go on. Suffice it to say that most importantly it is the wonderful volunteers and my red licorice and dark chocolate that also take me to my happy place.

Celebrations make me happy. Not only the ones that belong to my family, but also my dear friends. But being honest here, celebrations almost always make me sad. I always lose myself for some moments thinking about the possible potential celebrations I might not get to see. That part is frightening, as I said before I want more of everything. I will fight for it all. Each time I experience that wedding, moving up day or graduation, the birth of a new grandchild (or granddaughter since we now have six of them) or someone's birthday it makes me happy. I really do want it all.

My cancerversary makes me happy. For my fifth cancerversary we celebrated that milestone. I did my most favorite thing. We went on vacation with our family. We went on a cruise and had the best time. There is no better happy place then being with family. But believe me it is not easy to get six children and their children together at one time. This year when I started number nine we moved my mom up from Florida. Ninety-three years young, but it makes me happy to have her nearby so I can see her every week, but most importantly she gets to see her grandchildren and great grandchildren.

In November we will again do a trip to celebrate number ten.
The process is crazy but I have the will to get it done. This year we are heading to a ranch in upstate NY. I will have three full days to enjoy the family. Number ten will make me way more than happy, I will be ecstatic. Then I can start planning cancerversary fifteen. All celebrations I know can take us to our happy places.

In case you haven't realized it by now, simply said, my happiest place in the world is with my family.... especially my husband, children and grandchildren as well as the rest of the family and my friends. **It all comes down to the people.**

Family, family family

And I have a big one. Between my husband and me we have six children, wives and husbands, children and grandchildren that go along with them. They are my life's goal. I want more weddings, more grandchildren, more bat mitzvahs and simply more family time together.

I make the decisions of how I handle and share my cancer journey in my own way and on my own time. My husband is a rock and couldn't be more supportive. I try not to sweat the little stuff, but life happens. But if I am honest here, and that was the purpose of putting my thoughts on paper, he lost his wife to breast cancer not long before we met. Then on our first anniversary I was diagnosed. Not such good luck. We talk over all medical decisions. It is my instinct to protect him a little so there are times I keep emotions to myself. He comes to the important appointments and I tell him when it is not needed. My decision, my prerogative. Many times he just knows and hugs always come in handy. Did I mention sleeping pills at night also come in handy? I learned a long time ago the extra cancer demons and emotions come out just when you are closing your eyes.

The children are another issue. Mine are all adults and have a basic sense of everything. They know about trials; they generally know when I am going for scans. And of course the highs and lows of my ca125. Sometimes I send that group email to eleven people with an update, good or bad and sometimes I just don't feel like it. I may live with this cancer every day and deal with it every day, but it is not how I choose for my children to live their lives. And because of how well I feel and of course since I play my golf, work full time, play some tennis etc., I think they get to see a very positive, very living her life mom.

It doesn't mean that it doesn't come with some disappointments. Gonna be honest here as well. I don't believe there are perfect children or perfect people. We all have flaws. Sometimes I know they know about a scan and they don't ask, or they know my treatment is postponed and don't check on it. Here's what I've learned. If something is really important to me and I want them to ask or do something, I better damn well tell them. They are not mind readers and can't possibly know what I am thinking. They don't know when I get all the results or when I haven't kept them informed. To harbor a disappointment when I have control of my medical information and updates and how I myself have structured it is all on me. I make my choices and I hope I have taught them to do that as well. And I never, never for a minute doubt their love.

Recently a new friend and I talked at the Cancer Center. We discussed how we both did our treatments alone. We liked it that way. We didn't want to entertain. We wanted our families to have their normal days, (unless of course we had Benadryl and we needed rides home). We knew we had amazing support, but we also chose to protect the ones we love the most.

Grandchildren....how to deal with the cancer here is more specifically based upon age. For infants and toddlers, it is a non-issue, they are not going to understand, nor would I want them to. For my older ones (12 and 10), suffice it to say they know more now than they did before. How much exactly they know and when they know it is up to their parents. When we were at the San Diego zoo with the big girls, we decided that there was going to be a certain amount of walking, hills and sun. I was a little tired so maybe it made sense that we rented a wheelchair. I have a hard time with uphills. Doesn't affect my golf of course since I played the previous day, but hills are problematic at times.

The girls asked how come, and the answer was simple, just in case I got tired from some of the walking. Simple answer. The conversation was over before it started and we just proceeded through the zoo with me hopping out whenever I chose.

Everyone has different relationships with families and has the ability to handle it in the way you choose. What is right for some may not be right for others. You have the right and so do your families to tell you if it should be handled differently. I think I will leave the family section open to more thought and reflection since it is such a unique part of the journey we are all taking.

Living and Dying

I was going to leave this section blank since fortunately for me I have not had to deal with the issues related to end of life. I have covered my experience living with cancer. The end of life is a different story. I feel compelled that although I haven't had to discuss this or make decisions I want this story to be complete with as much information as I can come up with.

Most recently as I prepare for my upcoming trial (this is a story which doesn't end), I have begun taking some steps which I have never dealt with in the time since my original diagnosis. I know the side effects of this trial can be severe and I know there have been deaths. Different from when I started looking into it three years ago. The good news here is that because it is phase 1, I will be receiving a reduced dose. Yet, I feel compelled to make some preparations as necessary. I updated my will which I had last done almost ten years ago preparing for my first surgery. I am cleaning and straightening out things in my office and meeting with appropriate people to have difficult conversations. These are not just about life or death issues, they are also about the ability to get my job done efficiently. I feel it is important to have some back up plans in place. At minimum, I will be out of the office two weeks. Hopefully the maximum won't be longer. Yet as the person in charge I want to be responsible so I will prepare for what I can.

I think all people living with cancer spend time thinking about what happens when everything shuts down and treatment is not effective. This is the sadness we feel and the fear we live with.

So, although there is no plan and I hope to begin planning my 15th cancerversary after we pass 10 this year, I, like everyone else, have thought about it. I believe and heard so many thoughts on my discussion threads. I strongly believe this is fundamentally our decision. I know friends and family will want us to be a constant in their lives and to continue the fight. I have experienced so much over these years that I believe I will recognize when it is time for the game to end. I know my team of doctors will be forthright and will provide me with honest, realistic input. It is then I will know what to do. No funny punch line I can think of to end this section with so I will just let it go...

Playing it Forward

I have never had any interest in keeping a journal or a diary (at least in my adult life; not so much when I was young either). When I was diagnosed someone mentioned that it might help to write down my feelings and thoughts. I was pretty sure that I really had no interest in that. To me writing has always been a chore. Up until I wrote the piece for 'Friday's Corner' it was not an interest of mine. To be honest, there were plenty of nights when I was lying in bed when I knew there was so much information I could pass on, but I just had zero interest in taking the time to write. I could do it in my brain, I could talk it through and think of topics, but I didn't want to take the effort to write. I really have never, never liked writing!

But one piece and the ease at which it came to me changed my perspective. I am so fortunate to have so many wonderful people in my life. I am so fortunate for now to have a life living with this disease. I work, I play, I live. So the message here became simple. It was truly time to formally take the information I have learned and any expertise I have garnered and provide it for anyone and everyone who it might help. Cancer is cancer. The specifics are unique to each one but the experiences certainly overlap. This is my journey, the good, the bad and the better than ok. My education won't end nor will my fight.

If you or someone you know have additional questions, simply email me at: bringiton2255@gmail.com

All the proceeds from this book will go to Comfort Project 360 and the Ovarian Cancer Research Fund Alliance.

By working together we can make our lives just a little bit easier and I am happy to help in any way possible.

Cathy

RESOURCES:

Inspire.com – for a multitude of cancers
Facingourrisk.org – for BRCA positive information (Force)
Clinicaltrials.gov – for information on clinical trials
Every specific cancer has their own website
https://app.emergingmed.com/cancerstudylocator-Inspire/home -
locate trials

APPENDIX #1

WHEN YOU EXPECT OR RECEIVE A DIAGNOSIS

Questions to ask:
How soon are they doing a scan?
How long do they need to wait for scan results or could they get a wet read sooner?
What is Cancer type?
What is Staging? Metastasis?
Remember that no matter what the staging is – do not panic. Sometimes the level doesn't matter.
Although it is important, what is crucial is getting treatments that are effective. I am stage 3c out of 4. I am 1 step away. I've got 9 1/2 years of lots of different treatments. I know people who have passed with stage 2 or 3a. Much of your life depends on finding what is successful. There are truly impressive doctors around - never settle.
Exactly what did scan show?
What is the recommended treatment?
There are many options out there: Surgery, Chemo; new immunotherapies, radiation etc. Or combination of above. How soon can something be started is also a consideration.
Be cognizant of options in the NY area [or the area where you are]. You might or might not want a second opinion.
I stayed with one opinion at Barnabas because basically the protocol was the same all over. That isn't true with all cancers. Currently I have a team made up of doctors at Sloan, Dana Farber in Boston and U Penn. You go where you have the best recommendations for success, even if it is not your current facility.
What is the background of the doctor you are seeing?
Is he a general practitioner; oncologist?
Does the patient need a surgeon?
Oncology groups are sometime a general practice. Cancer Centers usually have oncologists with a specialty. That might have an influence on the doctors you choose.
What are the clinical trials which exist for the cancer or staging?
Are there any at the local hospital; what about in the city; are they having any success with new protocols?
Do research on clinicaltrials.gov site. Stay away from things that are

not reliable. Once you know what type of cancer, see if *Team Inspire* has a discussion group. This is an organization that has different cancer groups. You can ask any questions and people, generally person with cancer or family member will respond. Amazing source for information. They are already living it.

Make sure the hospital and/or doctors take all of your insurance.

Be the best advocates you can be.

Do due diligence when making decisions. When time is of the essence make sure information is gathered efficiently and succinctly.

APPENDIX #2

How to navigate the hundreds and hundreds of trials.

1. If you think you want to do a trial first thing to do is ask your Dr. Even if you have just been diagnosed, there are trials that deal with frontline treatment. Some hospitals have lots of trials and some none. Ask the question. Your Dr. may be able to recommend someone who can guide you if they can't. If you have used more than one Dr. question them all on potential trials.

2. Try and do a search on Clinicaltrials.gov. You are not expected to understand everything there. If you have talked about a drug with your Dr., then you can look up that drug in an area close to you or a nearby treatment center.

3. Reach out to names of people you can locate that are affiliated with the trial. Tell them your history and experience and see if they will send you what is called the consent form. You are not going to sign anything before you meet with dr but this form will describe the trial in detail. If you do commit to the trial this is the form you will have to sign in order to participate.

4. If you have participated in any on line support groups, ask a questions about potential trials. These are like minded cancer patients and cumulatively they can provide you with knowledge not simply acquired.

5. Don't get discouraged if you can't find an appropriate trial. Your Dr.

will provide you with recommendations for standard treatment.

APPENDIX # 3

Preprinted list for when you go to Doctor appointments away from your home treatment center:

MEDICAL HISTORY FORM

What medications are you currently taking?

Name   Dose   How often

What surgeries have you had: (this can be extensive for some)

Who is your primary dr?

Are there additional Doctors you would you like your records sent to?
Name, fax number

What other medical issues are you experiencing

This may not eliminate the check off form you have to fill out, but you won't necessarily have to keep repeating all the information that you include on this form.

Wouldn't it be nice to hand this off and just say "see attached".

Acknowledgements

Throughout this story I have thanked the many medical personnel, friends and family who have supported me through this journey.

I have to thank my wonderful friend and my editor Karen Cherins; I couldn't have completed this without your assistance and encouragement, with or without tracking. Thank you!

50984924R00033

Made in the USA
Middletown, DE
06 November 2017